A Foundational Guide to What Glucose is and Why it Matters...

GLUCOSE EXPLAINED

THE SERIES

Glucose Basics:
Understanding Blood Sugar
for Everyday Health

GET INFORMED

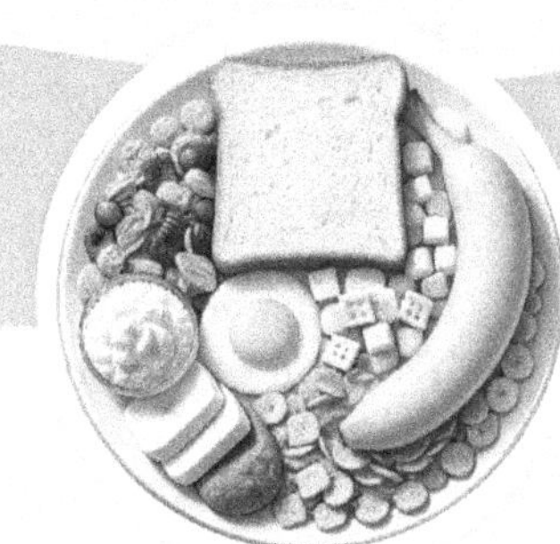

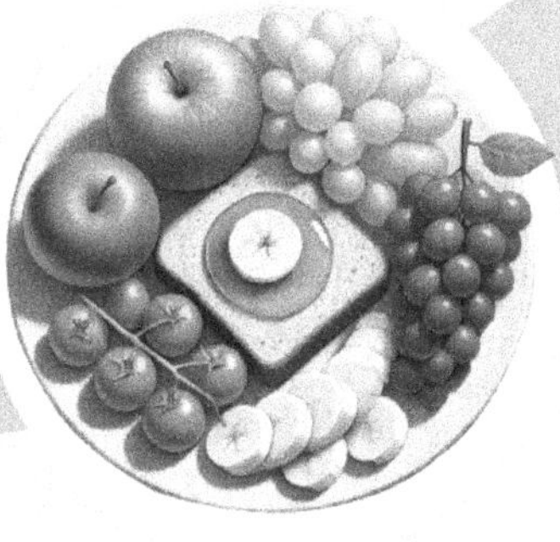

Darius Smith

Glucose Basics: Understanding Blood Sugar for Everyday Health

From the Series - Glucose Explained

TABLE OF CONTENT

CHAPTER 1:

WHAT IS GLUCOSE?

Exploring the Role of Glucose in Your Body

Glucose as Your Body's Fuel
Glucose is the body's preferred energy source, much like gasoline fuels a car. Just as a car won't run without gas, your body won't function without a sufficient supply of glucose. When you eat foods rich in carbohydrates, your body breaks them down into glucose, which enters the bloodstream. From there, glucose fuels everything from physical movement to mental activity. Even when you're resting or sleeping, glucose is powering critical functions like breathing and maintaining your heartbeat. Think of glucose as the currency your body uses to pay for all of its energetic needs—whether you're running a marathon or simply reading a book.

How Glucose Reaches Your Cells
The process of glucose reaching your cells is highly orchestrated, with insulin playing the

role of a "gatekeeper." After you eat, glucose enters your bloodstream, and this signals your pancreas to release insulin. Insulin works like a key, unlocking the doors of your cells so glucose can enter and be used as energy. Without insulin, glucose would stay in the bloodstream and could not get into the cells where it's needed. This is like having a bunch of groceries delivered to your house but no key to open the door and bring them inside. Insulin allows glucose to enter the house— your cells—so it can be "unpacked" and used.

How Glucose Powers Your Brain Your brain is a glucose powerhouse, consuming up to 20% of the body's energy, despite accounting for only 2% of its weight. This is because brain cells, called neurons, are constantly firing, even when you're at rest. Glucose is the primary fuel for neurons, and without enough of it, your brain can't function optimally. Have you ever felt mentally foggy or irritable when you're hungry? That's your brain signaling it's running low on glucose. It's like trying to work on a computer with a dying battery—tasks take longer, and your system slows down. Eating a small snack, particularly one containing carbohydrates, can often restore mental clarity within minutes.

Muscle Activity and Glucose
Glucose also plays a critical role in muscle function. During physical activity, your muscles rely on glucose to fuel movement. When you begin to exercise, the glucose stored in your muscles is rapidly broken down to provide energy. Think of it like revving up an engine—the faster you go, the more fuel you need. This is why athletes often eat carbohydrate-rich foods before a big race or game—they're essentially stocking up on glucose to ensure their muscles have enough fuel to perform at their best. But glucose isn't just important for athletes; even everyday activities like walking, cleaning, or gardening rely on glucose to keep you moving.

What Happens When Glucose Runs Low?
When your glucose levels dip too low, the effects can be swift and uncomfortable. This condition, known as hypoglycemia, often leads to feelings of dizziness, weakness, and even confusion. Imagine trying to drive a car on an empty gas tank—your body slows

down, and essential functions struggle to keep up. In response, the body has a built-in system to correct low glucose levels: the liver releases stored glucose to bring your levels back up. It's like having an emergency fuel reserve in your car. If your glucose levels remain low, though, you may need to refuel quickly with food. For instance, a piece of fruit or a handful of nuts can help restore normal glucose levels.

The Impact of Excess Glucose on the Body
Just as too little glucose can cause issues, too much glucose in your system also poses problems. When you consistently consume more glucose than your body needs, the excess is stored as fat. Think of this like a pantry that's overstocked with food—it's great to have supplies, but at a certain point, things start to spill over, making a mess. In the case of your body, this "spillover" can lead to weight gain and increase your risk of developing health issues like Type 2 diabetes. Excess glucose in the bloodstream also puts stress on your blood vessels and organs, potentially leading to complications like cardiovascular disease over time.

Glucose Storage: The Body's Backup System
When your body has more glucose than it needs immediately, it stores the extra in the liver and muscles in the form of glycogen. Think of glycogen as a "backup battery." When you're not eating, such as during sleep or between meals, your body taps into these reserves to maintain stable energy levels. This is especially useful for endurance activities or fasting periods. Your body essentially has a reserve tank it can pull from when glucose intake slows down. However, the storage space is limited. Once your liver and muscles are full of glycogen, any excess glucose is converted to fat for long-term storage.

The Role of Glucose in Healing and Recovery

Glucose isn't just about energy—it also plays a vital role in healing. When your body experiences physical stress, such as illness or injury, it needs more glucose to support the repair process. Just like how a construction site requires extra materials to rebuild, your body uses glucose as one of the primary fuels for healing tissues and fighting off infections. During recovery periods, the body's glucose demands increase, making it essential to maintain balanced blood sugar levels to support the healing process. This is one reason why people recovering from surgery or illness are often encouraged to eat nourishing, energy-dense foods.

Balancing Glucose for Optimal Health
Maintaining the right balance of glucose in your body is like keeping a well-oiled machine running smoothly. If glucose levels are too high or too low, it can throw your system off balance, leading to a range of health problems. Regular meals, a balanced diet, and physical activity all contribute to keeping your glucose levels in check. Just like maintaining a car, where you need to monitor oil levels, fuel, and tire pressure, balancing glucose requires regular attention to diet, exercise, and overall lifestyle choices. By being mindful of how much and what kind of food you eat, you can help ensure your glucose levels stay in a healthy range.

Glucose and Aging: A Lifelong Relationship
As we age, our relationship with glucose

shifts. Metabolism naturally slows down, which can affect how efficiently the body processes glucose. This is one reason why older adults are more susceptible to conditions like diabetes and high blood sugar. However, staying physically active and eating a diet rich in whole foods can help maintain healthy glucose levels even as you age. Think of it like an old car that still runs well because it's been carefully maintained over the years. With the right care and attention, you can keep your body's glucose system functioning optimally throughout your life.

How to Keep Glucose Levels Stable
Maintaining stable glucose levels is essential for preventing energy crashes, mood swings, and long-term health problems. One of the most effective ways to keep glucose stable is to eat regular, balanced meals that combine carbohydrates, proteins, and fats. For example, instead of eating a bag of chips as a snack, opt for an apple with peanut butter. The fiber in the apple and the protein in the peanut butter will slow the release of glucose into your bloodstream, providing sustained energy instead of a quick spike and crash.

Think of it like fueling a campfire: a mix of kindling and larger logs will keep the fire burning steadily for hours.

By understanding how glucose works in your body, you can make better choices to support long-term health and well-being. Whether it's fueling your brain, powering your muscles, or aiding in recovery, glucose is a vital part of the body's daily operations—one that deserves your attention and care.

CHAPTER 2:

HOW YOUR BODY PROCESSES GLUCOSE

Understanding Glucose Metabolism and Its Importance for Energy

What Is Glucose Metabolism? Glucose metabolism is the process by which your body converts food into energy. Think of it as a factory that takes raw materials, like carbohydrates, and turns them into fuel that powers your body's systems. After eating, carbohydrates are broken down into glucose, which is absorbed into the bloodstream. From there, glucose is either used immediately for energy or stored for later use. The process is like how your smartphone stores battery power—it either uses the charge immediately to run apps or saves energy for when it's needed most.

The Journey of Glucose in the Body Once glucose enters your bloodstream, it has two primary destinations: it can be used by cells for immediate energy, or it can be stored for later. Think of glucose as a delivery driver. When you eat, the "driver" picks up glucose and delivers it to your muscles, brain, and other organs. If you're physically active, your muscles will accept the delivery and use it right away to keep you moving. If you're at rest, glucose may be stored in your liver or muscles as glycogen for future use. It's a system that ensures energy is always available when needed.

The Role of Insulin in Glucose Metabolism
Insulin is a hormone produced by the pancreas that acts like a key, unlocking cells so glucose can enter and be used for energy. Imagine glucose is trying to enter a house (your cells), but the door is locked. Insulin is the key that opens the door, allowing glucose to come inside and fuel your body. Without insulin, glucose would remain in the bloodstream, leading to high blood sugar levels, which can cause long-term health issues. This careful balance between glucose and insulin is essential for maintaining stable energy levels and overall health.

How Your Body Converts Glucose into Energy

The actual process of converting glucose into energy occurs within your cells, specifically in an area called the mitochondria. The mitochondria are often referred to as the "powerhouses" of the cell because they take glucose and oxygen and convert them into a form of energy called ATP (adenosine triphosphate). This is the fuel that powers everything from your heartbeat to your ability to think and move. Think of mitochondria as a factory assembly line: glucose is the raw material, and ATP is the finished product, ready to be used by your body.

How Your Body Stores Glucose for Later

When your body has more glucose than it needs immediately, it stores the excess as glycogen. The liver and muscles are the main storage centers for glycogen. It's like putting money into a savings account—you're setting aside energy for times when you need it later, like during a workout or when you haven't eaten in a while. However, just like a savings account, there's a limit to how much glycogen can be stored. Once those storage tanks are full, any excess glucose gets converted into fat. This is why overeating, especially sugary foods, can lead to weight gain over time.

The Importance of Glucose for Energy
Glucose is your body's primary source of energy, particularly for the brain and muscles. If you've ever skipped a meal and felt light-headed, sluggish, or unable to focus, that's your body signaling a lack of glucose. Think of glucose as the gasoline that powers a car's engine. Without enough fuel, the car sputters and eventually stops. Your body works similarly—without sufficient glucose, your energy levels drop, and basic functions slow down. That's why it's important to maintain stable blood sugar levels by eating balanced meals that provide a steady release of glucose.

The Impact of Exercise on Glucose Metabolism
Exercise plays a vital role in how your body uses glucose. When you exercise, your muscles require more energy, so they use the glucose available in your bloodstream and stored in your muscles as glycogen. It's like

using extra electricity during peak hours—the more active you are, the more energy (glucose) your body consumes. Regular physical activity improves your body's sensitivity to insulin, meaning glucose can be used more efficiently. Think of exercise as a tune-up for your metabolic system, helping it run smoothly and preventing glucose from building up in your bloodstream.

What Happens When Glucose Metabolism Is Disrupted?

When glucose metabolism isn't working properly, it can lead to health problems like insulin resistance or diabetes. In insulin resistance, your body doesn't respond as well to insulin, meaning glucose stays in the bloodstream instead of entering cells. It's like trying to unlock a door with a key that no longer fits—it becomes harder and harder to let glucose in. Over time, this can lead to chronically high blood sugar levels, which may cause damage to your blood vessels, nerves, and organs. Managing your diet and exercise habits is key to preventing disruptions in glucose metabolism.

Balancing Glucose for Optimal Performance

Keeping your blood sugar levels stable is crucial for maintaining optimal energy levels throughout the day. Eating small, frequent meals that include complex carbohydrates, fiber, and healthy fats can help regulate glucose levels. For example, instead of grabbing a sugary snack that causes a quick spike in glucose, opt for whole grains or nuts, which provide a more sustained release of energy. It's like choosing slow-burning logs for a fire instead of kindling that flares up and dies down quickly. The goal is to create a steady, even burn—fueling your body without dramatic rises and falls in blood sugar.

How Stress Affects Glucose Metabolism

When you're stressed, your body releases hormones like cortisol and adrenaline, which can affect glucose metabolism. These hormones trigger your liver to release stored glucose into the bloodstream, providing a burst of energy to help you deal with the stressor. This response is part of the "fight or flight" mechanism, designed to give you the energy needed to escape danger. However, in today's world, most stressors don't require physical action, so this extra glucose often goes unused, leading to elevated blood sugar levels. Managing stress through relaxation techniques like meditation or deep breathing can help keep your glucose metabolism balanced.

The Role of Diet in Glucose Metabolism
What you eat plays a huge role in how efficiently your body metabolizes glucose. Foods high in refined sugars, like candy and soda, cause rapid spikes in blood sugar, followed by sharp crashes. It's like pouring lighter fluid on a fire—it flares up dramatically but burns out quickly. On the other hand, complex carbohydrates, found in foods like vegetables, whole grains, and legumes, break down more slowly, providing a steady release of glucose. Think of these as slow-burning coals that keep your body energized over a longer period. Incorporating protein and healthy fats into your meals also helps slow down glucose absorption, promoting balanced blood sugar levels.

A Balanced Approach to Glucose Metabolism

To maintain healthy glucose metabolism, it's important to focus on a balanced lifestyle. Regular exercise, stress management, and a diet rich in whole foods all contribute to efficient glucose processing. For example, a combination of walking, yoga, or strength training can help improve insulin sensitivity, making it easier for your body to use glucose for energy. Similarly, reducing sugary snacks and incorporating more fiber-rich foods can prevent blood sugar spikes and crashes. Think of these changes as tuning your body's engine, ensuring that your metabolic system runs smoothly and efficiently.

Conclusion: Supporting Your Body's Glucose Needs

Understanding glucose metabolism helps you take control of your energy levels and overall health. By eating balanced meals, staying active, and managing stress, you can support your body's ability to efficiently process glucose, providing steady, sustainable energy throughout the day. When glucose metabolism functions well, your body can easily convert food into fuel, helping you feel more energized and focused, whether you're at work, exercising, or spending time with family. By making small, mindful choices, you can maintain a healthy balance of glucose and set the foundation for long-term wellness.

CHAPTER 3:

BLOOD SUGAR AND YOUR HEALTH

The Crucial Connection Between Glucose Levels and Wellness

Glucose: The Body's Preferred Energy Source

Glucose is the primary fuel that powers your body. Every cell relies on this simple sugar for energy, from your muscles to your brain. When glucose enters your bloodstream, it becomes available to be used as energy or stored for later use. But while glucose is essential, managing it is key. Think of glucose like fuel for a car. Too little, and the engine sputters; too much, and it can flood the system, causing damage over time. Achieving balance is what keeps the engine (your body) running smoothly and efficiently. Just as high or low fuel levels can affect performance, fluctuating glucose can impact everything from your mood to your ability to focus.

Glucose and Energy Regulation

You've probably noticed that after eating, you often feel energized or sleepy, depending on what you ate. This is because your glucose levels spike after meals, and how efficiently your body processes and manages this glucose directly impacts how you feel. Simple carbohydrates, like sugary snacks or processed foods, lead to quick spikes and crashes in glucose levels. This rollercoaster can leave you feeling sluggish or irritable. In contrast, complex carbohydrates like whole grains, paired with proteins and healthy fats, lead to a slower release of glucose, giving you a more sustained energy level. This connection between glucose and energy explains why certain foods make you feel great while others leave you in an afternoon slump.

The Role of Insulin in Glucose Management

Insulin is the hormone responsible for moving glucose from your bloodstream into cells where it can be used for energy. When everything functions properly, insulin maintains healthy glucose levels in a seamless dance. However, problems arise when the body's insulin production or its sensitivity to insulin falters. If the body can't produce enough insulin, or if cells become resistant to its effects, glucose builds up in the bloodstream, leading to high blood sugar. This is where the delicate balance between glucose and wellness begins to shift. For individuals with insulin resistance or diabetes, even small missteps in diet or activity can lead to significant imbalances, highlighting the importance of glucose regulation for overall health.

Glucose and Brain Health

Your brain is a glucose-hungry organ, consuming around 20% of your body's energy at rest. Stable glucose levels mean clearer thinking, better concentration, and improved memory. When your blood sugar levels dip too low, your brain's performance suffers. This can manifest as mental fog, difficulty focusing, or mood swings. On the other hand, chronic high glucose levels can damage blood vessels in the brain, contributing to cognitive decline and an increased risk of dementia. Think of glucose as the fuel that powers not just your body but your mind. Keeping your glucose levels stable is one of the best things you can do for long-term brain health.

The Impact of Glucose on Emotional Well-Being

Many people don't realize that glucose imbalances can affect more than just physical health—they can also influence mood and emotions. When glucose levels crash, so can your mood. You may feel anxious, irritable, or even depressed. These feelings often stem from the brain not getting enough energy to function optimally. Over time, chronic glucose imbalances can contribute to more significant emotional disturbances, making it harder to cope with stress or maintain a positive outlook. Conversely, maintaining steady glucose levels can help stabilize your mood and enhance emotional resilience, allowing you to feel more grounded and less prone to emotional highs and lows.

Glucose and Immune Function

Stable glucose levels are not just important for energy and mood; they also play a critical role in supporting your immune system. High blood sugar can suppress the immune response, making it harder for your body to fight off infections. It can also contribute to chronic inflammation, which is linked to a variety of diseases, from heart disease to cancer. Keeping glucose levels within a healthy range helps to bolster your immune system, reduce inflammation, and prevent the onset of illness. A well-balanced glucose level is like giving your immune system the tools it needs to function at its best.

The Long-Term Health Risks of Glucose Imbalance

Over time, unmanaged glucose levels can lead to serious long-term health consequences. Chronic high blood sugar levels contribute to conditions like type 2 diabetes, heart disease, stroke, and nerve damage. On the other end of the spectrum, frequent low blood sugar can cause dizziness, fainting, and long-term cognitive issues. The importance of keeping glucose balanced cannot be overstated. It's not just about avoiding short-term discomfort; it's about preventing long-term damage that can impact your quality of life. Think of maintaining glucose levels like tending to a garden—regular care and attention prevent weeds (or diseases) from taking root and damaging the ecosystem (your body).

Building Sustainable Habits for Glucose Wellness

The good news is that managing your glucose levels and overall wellness doesn't have to be overwhelming. Small, consistent changes in your diet, activity levels, and stress management can make a significant difference. Start by incorporating more whole foods, reducing processed sugars, and focusing on balanced meals that combine proteins, healthy fats, and complex carbohydrates. Regular physical activity, even light exercise like walking, helps your body use glucose more efficiently. And don't underestimate the power of stress management techniques like mindfulness or deep breathing—stress hormones can cause glucose spikes, disrupting the balance. By developing these habits, you're not just improving your glucose levels today; you're setting yourself up for a lifetime of better health.

Conclusion: Why Glucose Wellness Matters for Overall Health

Understanding the connection between glucose and wellness is essential for anyone looking to improve their health. Glucose is at the heart of how your body functions, impacting everything from your energy and mood to your long-term health. By managing glucose levels effectively, you can enhance not only your physical health but also your mental and emotional well-being. The journey to glucose balance is about making small, sustainable changes that lead to big results over time. When you take control of your glucose, you take control of your wellness.

CHAPTER 4:

INSULIN: YOUR GLUCOSE REGULATOR

How Insulin Helps Balance Blood Sugar in Your System

The Key Role of Insulin in Blood Sugar Regulation

Insulin is often referred to as the body's "blood sugar manager" because its primary role is to help regulate glucose levels. It acts like a traffic cop, directing glucose where it needs to go and making sure everything flows smoothly. Produced by the pancreas, insulin is released when you eat, particularly when you consume carbohydrates, which are broken down into glucose. The goal is simple: insulin ensures that glucose gets into your cells where it can be used as energy, or stored for later use. Without this vital hormone, glucose would accumulate in the bloodstream, causing high blood sugar levels.

How Insulin Functions as a Key to Unlock Your Cells

Imagine glucose as a guest trying to enter a locked house, which in this case is your cell. Insulin acts as the key to open the door, allowing glucose to enter and provide energy. When you eat, your blood sugar levels rise, signaling the pancreas to release insulin. This insulin binds to receptors on the surface of your cells, unlocking them so glucose can move from the bloodstream into the cell. Once inside, glucose is either used immediately for energy or stored as glycogen for later use. Without insulin, glucose can't access the cells, leading to a build-up in the bloodstream, much like a keyless guest standing outside a locked door.

How Your Body Knows When to Release Insulin

Your body is an incredible system that constantly monitors blood sugar levels. As soon as glucose enters your bloodstream after a meal, specialized cells in the pancreas, called beta cells, detect this rise. This is like your body's internal thermostat—it senses when glucose levels are too high and signals the release of insulin to bring them back into balance. This finely tuned process ensures that your blood sugar stays within a safe range, preventing both highs (hyperglycemia) and lows (hypoglycemia). For instance, after a meal rich in carbohydrates, insulin is released to ensure your cells absorb the sugar, but when you haven't eaten for a while, the pancreas holds off on insulin release to avoid depleting glucose levels.

Balancing Immediate Energy Needs and Future Storage

Insulin doesn't just shuttle glucose into cells for immediate energy; it also plays a crucial role in deciding when to store excess glucose. Picture your body as a household budget system. When you have extra income (glucose), some of it goes towards immediate expenses (your energy needs), and the rest is saved in a bank account (glycogen stores in the liver and muscles) for future use. When you've eaten more carbohydrates than your body needs at the moment, insulin signals the liver and muscles to store the excess glucose as glycogen. Later, when blood sugar levels drop, this glycogen can be converted back into glucose to keep your energy levels stable.

What Happens When Insulin Sensitivity Decreases

Insulin sensitivity refers to how responsive your cells are to insulin's signals. In a healthy system, your cells respond quickly and efficiently, absorbing glucose as soon as insulin binds to them. However, over time, factors such as poor diet, inactivity, and excess weight can reduce your cells' sensitivity to insulin. Think of it as the door to your cell becoming rusty; even though insulin is there, it can't unlock the door as easily, meaning glucose can't enter as effectively. This leads to higher blood sugar levels because glucose is stuck in the bloodstream. The pancreas compensates by producing even more insulin, but over time, this can wear down the system, potentially leading to insulin resistance or type 2 diabetes.

How to Improve Insulin Sensitivity

The good news is that insulin sensitivity can be improved with lifestyle changes. Regular physical activity, for example, is one of the most effective ways to enhance how your body responds to insulin. When you exercise, your muscles use glucose for energy, reducing the amount of insulin needed to transport glucose into cells. It's like lubricating the door hinges, making it easier for insulin to do its job. In addition to exercise, a balanced diet rich in fiber and low in refined sugars helps prevent large spikes in blood sugar, easing the workload on insulin. Consider focusing on whole grains, lean proteins, and healthy fats, which help maintain a steady release of glucose and keep insulin working efficiently.

How Stress and Sleep Impact Insulin Function

You might be surprised to learn that stress and poor sleep can significantly affect how insulin works in your body. When you're stressed, your body releases hormones like cortisol and adrenaline, which trigger the release of glucose into your bloodstream as part of the "fight or flight" response. While this extra glucose is helpful if you need to react quickly in a dangerous situation, chronic stress can lead to consistently elevated blood sugar levels, forcing your pancreas to work overtime producing insulin. Sleep deprivation has a similar effect. Without enough rest, your body's ability to manage blood sugar deteriorates, and insulin sensitivity decreases, making it harder to balance your blood sugar.

The Connection Between Diet and Insulin Efficiency

The types of food you eat directly impact how well insulin can balance your blood sugar. Diets high in refined carbohydrates and sugars can overwhelm the pancreas with a constant need for insulin production, leading to what's called "insulin overproduction." When you consume sugary foods, they're rapidly broken down into glucose, flooding your bloodstream and causing insulin to rush in to manage the spike. This frequent insulin demand can eventually tire out your pancreas, leading to inefficiencies in blood sugar regulation. On the flip side, diets rich in whole foods like vegetables, legumes, and healthy fats provide a slower release of glucose into the bloodstream, giving insulin the time it needs to do its job effectively.

Why Consistency in Blood Sugar Levels Matters

One of insulin's most important tasks is keeping your blood sugar levels within a narrow, safe range. Large fluctuations in blood sugar can lead to feeling jittery, irritable, or fatigued. Insulin prevents these ups and downs by ensuring that glucose is absorbed steadily after meals. Think of it as maintaining a steady fuel flow to an engine; if too much or too little fuel is provided, the engine sputters. Your body works best when there is a consistent supply of glucose. Insulin plays the central role in maintaining this balance, keeping you energized and alert throughout the day.

The Role of Insulin in Preventing High and Low Blood Sugar

Insulin's balancing act is crucial in preventing two dangerous conditions: hyperglycemia (high blood sugar) and hypoglycemia (low blood sugar). If too much glucose remains in the bloodstream due to insufficient insulin, hyperglycemia can develop, leading to symptoms such as increased thirst, frequent urination, and fatigue. If left untreated, chronic hyperglycemia can damage your organs, nerves, and blood vessels. On the other hand, if insulin removes too much glucose from your bloodstream, hypoglycemia can occur. This condition can cause dizziness, confusion, and even loss of consciousness if not addressed promptly. Insulin, therefore, acts like a thermostat, constantly adjusting to keep your blood sugar within the optimal range.

How Insulin and Glucagon Work Together
While insulin works to lower blood sugar by storing glucose, another hormone called glucagon plays the opposite role. When your blood sugar levels drop too low—such as between meals or during exercise—glucagon signals the liver to release stored glycogen, which is then converted back into glucose and released into the bloodstream. This teamwork between insulin and glucagon keeps your blood sugar from getting too high or too low, ensuring that your body always has the right amount of energy available. Imagine it as a see-saw—when blood sugar rises, insulin steps in to bring it down, and when blood sugar falls, glucagon steps up to lift it back to normal levels.

The Importance of Long-Term Insulin Health

Maintaining insulin health over the long term is critical for preventing metabolic diseases like type 2 diabetes. As we've discussed, diet and lifestyle choices play a significant role in ensuring that your insulin continues to function optimally. Regular exercise, a diet low in processed foods, managing stress, and getting enough sleep are all powerful tools for keeping your insulin system in check. Think of these practices as preventive maintenance for your body—just as you would service your car regularly to avoid breakdowns, taking care of your insulin health today helps prevent more serious issues down the road.

Conclusion: Insulin as Your Blood Sugar Regulator

Insulin is much more than just a hormone—it's the key regulator of your body's energy system. By ensuring that glucose is absorbed by your cells and stored for later use, insulin keeps your blood sugar in check and provides you with the energy you need for daily activities. Understanding how insulin works gives you the power to make informed choices about your diet, exercise, and lifestyle, all of which contribute to healthy blood sugar levels. By supporting your insulin function, you can maintain consistent energy, avoid blood sugar swings, and lay the groundwork for long-term health.

CHAPTER 5:

WHAT HAPPENS WHEN GLUCOSE LEVELS SPIKE?

Recognizing the Risks of High Blood Sugar and Symptoms

What Is High Blood Sugar and Why Does It Matter?

High blood sugar, or hyperglycemia, occurs when there is too much glucose circulating in your bloodstream. While the term "high" may seem subjective, it refers to blood sugar levels that exceed the healthy range needed to maintain bodily function. Consistently elevated blood sugar is like having too much fuel in your car's tank—it can lead to severe problems if not managed properly. Unlike a one-time spike in blood sugar after a heavy meal, chronic high blood sugar levels can wear down your body over time, causing damage to vital organs and tissues. This is particularly concerning for individuals with diabetes or those at risk of developing it.

Understanding the Impact of Glucose on Your   Body

To grasp the risks of high blood sugar, think of glucose as your body's energy currency. When you eat, carbohydrates are broken down into glucose, which enters the bloodstream. Normally, insulin helps regulate this process, ensuring glucose is absorbed by cells for energy. However, when blood sugar levels remain high, the body is essentially flooded with excess glucose. Instead of being stored or used effectively, this glucose builds up in the bloodstream, causing stress to vital organs. It's akin to overwatering a plant—at first, the plant may thrive, but eventually, too much water drowns it, leading to irreversible damage. This is how high blood sugar can eventually harm your heart, kidneys, eyes, and   nerves.

Common Symptoms of High Blood Sugar

Recognizing the symptoms of high blood sugar can be challenging because they may seem ordinary or overlap with other conditions. Common symptoms include frequent urination, excessive thirst, unexplained weight loss, and fatigue. Imagine your body as a sponge. When blood sugar levels are high, the sponge (your body) becomes overwhelmed and tries to squeeze out excess water (glucose). This causes the kidneys to work harder, resulting in frequent trips to the bathroom and constant thirst. Fatigue occurs because your cells aren't getting the energy they need from glucose, leaving you feeling drained even after a good night's sleep. Other symptoms include blurred vision, headaches, and slow-healing wounds, all signs that your body is struggling to manage the overload of glucose.

Frequent Urination: Your Body's Warning Signal

One of the earliest signs of high blood sugar is frequent urination. The kidneys, which filter blood, react to high glucose levels by trying to flush out the excess through urine. This process can be compared to a coffee filter that is overfilled—just as water quickly passes through an overloaded filter, excess glucose is expelled through urine when the kidneys are overburdened. The body's constant need to rid itself of glucose leads to increased urination, which can become particularly noticeable at night. If you find yourself waking up repeatedly to use the bathroom, it may be a sign that your blood sugar levels are too high. This constant flushing also leads to dehydration, as the body loses more fluids than it takes in.

Excessive Thirst: A Consequence of Dehydration

Because frequent urination causes dehydration, excessive thirst soon follows. The body, having lost significant amounts of water through urine, tries to compensate by making you feel parched. This thirst isn't like the usual dryness you experience after a workout; it feels insatiable, no matter how much water you drink. The connection between thirst and dehydration due to high blood sugar is simple: the more glucose your kidneys filter out, the more water they need to carry that glucose away. The resulting thirst is your body's desperate plea for hydration. If you notice you're drinking far more fluids than usual but still feel thirsty, it's a sign that you should check your blood sugar levels.

Unexplained Weight Loss: When Your Body Can't Use Glucose Properly
One of the more puzzling symptoms of high blood sugar is unexplained weight loss. You might think high blood sugar would lead to weight gain due to an excess of energy in the bloodstream, but the opposite can occur. When your cells can't absorb glucose because of insulin resistance or insufficient insulin production, your body starts breaking down fat and muscle to use as energy. It's like trying to run a car without gasoline; in the absence of fuel (glucose), your body turns to alternative sources, leading to weight loss. While this might sound like a good thing, it's actually dangerous. The weight loss occurs because your body is essentially starving, unable to access the glucose it needs to function.

Fatigue: Running on Empty
Fatigue is another common symptom of high blood sugar and can be one of the most debilitating. Despite having plenty of glucose in your bloodstream, your cells are essentially starved for energy because they can't absorb that glucose efficiently. Think of it like trying to

use a smartphone with no battery—your body has the tools (glucose) it needs but no way to access the energy. This constant state of low energy leaves you feeling tired, sluggish, and unable to focus. If you find yourself exhausted even after a full night's sleep, or you're unable to perform daily tasks without feeling worn out, it could be due to high blood sugar levels.

Blurred Vision: A Subtle Sign of Trouble
High blood sugar doesn't just affect how you feel—it can also impact how you see. When glucose levels rise, fluid can leak into the lens of the eye, causing it to swell and change shape. This is why many people with high blood sugar experience blurred vision. It's like looking through a camera lens that's out of focus—everything appears blurry or distorted. This issue often resolves once blood sugar levels are brought back under control, but if left unchecked, it can lead to more serious complications such as diabetic retinopathy, which can cause permanent vision loss. Paying attention to changes in your vision, even subtle ones, can be an early indicator that your blood sugar is too high.

Headaches and Difficulty Concentrating
Elevated blood sugar can also affect brain function, leading to headaches and difficulty concentrating. The brain relies on a steady supply of glucose to function properly. When blood sugar levels are too high or too low, cognitive function can be impaired. You may experience brain fog, where simple tasks become difficult, or you might have frequent headaches due to fluctuations in blood sugar. It's similar to the way low fuel levels can make a car sputter—the brain becomes sluggish without the right amount of glucose. If you find that you're having trouble focusing or frequently battling headaches, it may be worth examining your blood sugar levels.

Slow-Healing Wounds and Frequent Infections
Another often overlooked sign of high blood sugar is slow-healing wounds. When blood sugar levels are elevated, it can impair your body's ability to repair itself. Cuts, scrapes, and bruises take longer to heal because the excess glucose in your blood slows down the repair process. Additionally, high blood sugar weakens your immune system, making you

more susceptible to infections. Think of it as trying to fix a leaky faucet with sticky hands— everything takes longer and becomes more complicated. If you notice that your wounds are taking longer than usual to heal, or if you're frequently battling infections like yeast infections or urinary tract infections, it may be a sign of high blood sugar levels.

The Long-Term Risks of Ignoring High Blood Sugar

While occasional spikes in blood sugar aren't necessarily a cause for alarm, persistently high levels can lead to serious complications over time. Chronic high blood sugar damages blood vessels, which can affect the heart, kidneys, and nerves. This damage increases your risk for conditions like heart disease, kidney failure, and diabetic neuropathy, a type of nerve damage that causes pain and numbness, often in the legs and feet. Imagine a river constantly flooding its banks— eventually, the surrounding land becomes eroded and damaged. That's what happens to your body when blood sugar remains elevated. Taking steps to manage your blood sugar now can prevent these long-term complications.

How to Take Control of High Blood Sugar
The good news is that high blood sugar is manageable with the right lifestyle changes. Simple steps like eating a balanced diet, exercising regularly, and managing stress can help lower blood sugar and prevent complications. For example, regular exercise helps your muscles use glucose more efficiently, lowering your blood sugar naturally. Meanwhile, a diet rich in fiber and low in refined sugars helps maintain stable glucose levels throughout the day. Think of it like adjusting the flow of water in a garden—by making small tweaks to your diet and lifestyle, you can prevent the flood of high blood sugar and keep your body functioning optimally.

Conclusion: Don't Ignore the Warning Signs
Recognizing the risks and symptoms of high blood sugar is the first step towards preventing serious health complications. While it may be easy to dismiss symptoms like fatigue or frequent urination, they are often early warning signs that your body is

struggling to manage glucose. Paying attention to these signals and making necessary lifestyle changes can help protect you from the long-term effects of high blood sugar, such as heart disease, nerve damage, and vision problems. By understanding how high blood sugar affects your body and taking proactive steps to address it, you can maintain your health and prevent more serious issues down the line.

CHAPTER 6:

UNDERSTANDING HYPOGLYCEMIA

The Dangers of Low Blood Sugar and How to Manage It

What Is Low Blood Sugar? Low blood sugar, or hypoglycemia, occurs when glucose levels in your blood drop below the normal range. Glucose is your body's primary source of energy, and when you don't have enough of it, your body struggles to function. Imagine your body as a car, and glucose is the gasoline. When the fuel level gets too low, the car may stutter, slow down, or even stop altogether. This is exactly what happens to your body during hypoglycemia—it starts to malfunction because it doesn't have the fuel it needs to keep running. It's more common in people with diabetes, especially those who take insulin, but it can happen to anyone under certain conditions.

The Immediate Risks of Low Blood Sugar
When blood sugar drops too low, it can lead to

immediate, serious consequences. The brain, which relies heavily on glucose for energy, is particularly vulnerable. You may start to feel dizzy, confused, or disoriented. In more severe cases, people can faint, have seizures, or even go into a coma. Think of low blood sugar like a battery in your phone running dangerously low. First, your phone slows down, apps don't work as efficiently, and eventually, it shuts down. Similarly, when your glucose levels fall, your body and brain start to slow down, and if left unchecked, it could be life-threatening. It's vital to recognize the symptoms early and act quickly to prevent a medical emergency.

Recognizing Early Warning Signs
The symptoms of low blood sugar can come on suddenly, but recognizing them early can help you manage the situation before it becomes critical. Common symptoms include shakiness, sweating, irritability, hunger, and a rapid heartbeat. It's like your body's internal alarm system going off, warning you that it needs more energy. The shakiness you feel is similar to what happens when you haven't eaten for a long time; your muscles start to

tremble because they're not getting enough glucose. The sweating and rapid heartbeat are your body's way of activating your "fight or flight" response, a signal that it's running low on fuel and needs help. Understanding these signals is key to preventing more severe symptoms.

How Low Blood Sugar Affects Your Brain
Your brain consumes more glucose than any other part of your body. When blood sugar levels drop, the brain is the first organ to suffer. Initially, you may experience confusion, difficulty concentrating, or mood swings. These symptoms might feel like you're suddenly "foggy-headed" or irritable for no apparent reason. Imagine trying to use a computer that's lagging and struggling to process commands; this is what your brain is going through when it doesn't have enough glucose. If low blood sugar persists, these cognitive symptoms can escalate into more severe conditions like memory loss, dizziness, and eventually unconsciousness. For this reason, addressing low blood sugar quickly is crucial for mental clarity and overall safety.

The Long-Term Risks of Repeated Hypoglycemia

While the immediate effects of low blood sugar are alarming, repeated episodes can cause long-term damage, especially to your cardiovascular and nervous systems. Hypoglycemia can put extra strain on the heart, increasing your risk for arrhythmias or even heart attacks. Additionally, frequent low blood sugar episodes can dull your body's natural warning system, making it harder to recognize when your glucose is dropping in the future. It's like constantly turning down the volume on a fire alarm—you might not hear it when a real emergency happens. Over time, this "hypoglycemia unawareness" can leave you vulnerable to more dangerous episodes without your body giving you the proper warning signals.

Daily Habits That Contribute to Low Blood Sugar

There are several everyday factors that can cause your blood sugar to drop unexpectedly. Skipping meals or eating meals that are too small are among the most common culprits. Think of food as the "fuel stops" your body needs throughout the day. If you skip a meal, it's like trying to drive a long distance without stopping for gas—you'll eventually run out of energy. Exercising intensely without adjusting your carbohydrate intake can also lead to low blood sugar. Physical activity burns through glucose quickly, and without replenishing it, your blood sugar can drop to unsafe levels. Lastly, consuming alcohol, especially on an empty stomach, can cause delayed hypoglycemia as your liver prioritizes metabolizing the alcohol over releasing stored glucose.

Managing Low Blood Sugar in Daily Life
One of the most effective ways to manage low blood sugar is through balanced, regular eating habits. Eating smaller, more frequent meals throughout the day ensures that your body has a steady supply of glucose. It's like maintaining a slow, steady flow of gasoline to your car rather than waiting for the tank to run dry before refueling. Foods rich in complex carbohydrates—such as whole grains, fruits, and vegetables—are particularly beneficial because they release glucose gradually, providing a more sustained energy supply.

Incorporating protein and healthy fats into your meals can further stabilize your blood sugar levels, helping to prevent the spikes and crashes that lead to hypoglycemia.

Quick Fixes for Immediate Low Blood Sugar

If you find yourself in the midst of a hypoglycemic episode, acting fast is crucial. The most common recommendation is to follow the "15-15 rule"—consume 15 grams of fast-acting carbohydrates, then wait 15 minutes and check your blood sugar levels again. Examples of fast-acting carbs include glucose tablets, a half-cup of fruit juice, or a tablespoon of honey. These are simple sugars that your body can absorb quickly, raising your blood sugar in a matter of minutes. It's like adding a splash of fuel to your tank when you're running on empty—it gives you just enough energy to get back on track. However, be cautious not to overeat, as this can cause a blood sugar spike.

The Role of Medication in Hypoglycemia

Certain medications, particularly insulin and some oral diabetes drugs, can cause low blood sugar. If you're managing diabetes, it's essential to work with your healthcare provider to adjust your medication as needed to avoid hypoglycemia. Imagine your medication as a thermostat that controls the temperature in your home. If it's set too low, you'll feel cold (low blood sugar), and if it's set too high, the heat becomes unbearable (high blood sugar). Regularly monitoring your blood sugar and adjusting your insulin doses or medication under your doctor's guidance can help maintain that ideal "temperature," preventing dangerous drops in glucose levels.

Preventing Low Blood Sugar During Exercise

Exercise is an excellent way to manage blood sugar, but it requires careful planning if you're prone to hypoglycemia. Before you engage in physical activity, it's important to check your blood sugar levels and ensure they're in a safe range. Think of your body like a car preparing for a long road trip—you need to ensure there's enough fuel to get you through. Eating a small snack that contains both carbohydrates and protein before exercise can help prevent blood sugar from dropping during your workout. Additionally, you should keep a fast-acting carbohydrate, like a sports drink or glucose gel, on hand during exercise in case your blood sugar dips.

Balancing Diet and Blood Sugar for Long-Term Health

In the long run, managing low blood sugar is about maintaining balance in your diet and lifestyle. Incorporating foods that provide steady, sustained energy will help prevent the highs and lows that come with blood sugar fluctuations. It's helpful to think of your blood sugar like a wave—you want gentle, rolling waves rather than sharp peaks and crashes. Consistently eating balanced meals, staying hydrated, and getting regular, moderate exercise can keep your blood sugar levels stable. This balance reduces the risk of hypoglycemia while promoting overall health and well-being.

When to Seek Medical Help

While low blood sugar can often be managed at home, there are times when medical intervention is necessary. If you experience severe symptoms, such as seizures, unconsciousness, or persistent hypoglycemia that doesn't respond to food, it's crucial to seek emergency medical care. Just like a car running out of fuel on the highway, sometimes you need roadside assistance. In such cases, emergency services can provide intravenous glucose to quickly raise your blood sugar to safe levels. If you're experiencing frequent low blood sugar episodes, it's essential to speak with your healthcare provider to adjust your treatment plan and prevent future occurrences.

Conclusion: Taking Control of Low Blood Sugar

Understanding the dangers of low blood sugar and how to manage it effectively is key to maintaining both immediate and long-term health. By learning to recognize the early warning signs, making smart choices about your diet and exercise, and understanding the role of medication, you can take control of hypoglycemia before it controls you. Managing low blood sugar isn't just about preventing emergencies—it's about living a balanced, healthy life with the energy and focus you need to thrive.

CHAPTER 7:

GLUCOSE AND DIABETES: THE ESSENTIAL LINK

How Diabetes Affects Glucose and Long-Term Health Outcomes

Understanding Diabetes and Its Impact on Glucose

Diabetes is a chronic condition that fundamentally alters the way your body handles glucose. Glucose is the primary fuel source for your cells, but when you have diabetes, the body struggles to either produce or use insulin properly. Insulin acts as a key that unlocks cells, allowing glucose to enter and be used for energy. Without this process working efficiently, glucose builds up in the bloodstream, leading to high blood sugar levels. Imagine glucose as traffic in a city. When everything is running smoothly, traffic flows, and cars reach their destinations (your cells). In diabetes, however, it's like a major traffic jam—glucose can't get to where it needs to go, which creates chaos throughout your body.

Type 1 and Type 2 Diabetes: Different Paths, Same Outcome

Diabetes comes in two main forms: Type 1 and Type 2. Both types affect glucose regulation but in different ways. In Type 1 diabetes, the body's immune system mistakenly attacks insulin-producing cells in the pancreas. This leaves the body without enough insulin to regulate blood sugar levels. Think of it as a factory shutting down the production line for insulin—without it, glucose can't enter the cells. People with Type 1 diabetes rely on insulin injections to survive. On the other hand, Type 2 diabetes is more like the body's cells becoming resistant to insulin. The insulin is there, but it doesn't work as well, and the cells don't respond as they should. This form is often associated with lifestyle factors, such as diet, physical inactivity, and weight. Regardless of the type, the end result is the same: glucose builds up in the bloodstream, causing damage over time.

How High Blood Sugar Damages the Body

When glucose levels remain consistently high, it begins to affect various systems in your body. Over time, high blood sugar can damage blood vessels, leading to complications such as heart disease, stroke, and kidney failure. Imagine pouring sugary syrup through a straw every day. Eventually, the syrup will coat the inside of the straw, causing blockages and making it difficult for anything to flow through smoothly. This is similar to how high blood sugar thickens and damages blood vessels, making it harder for blood to circulate. The small blood vessels in your eyes, kidneys, and extremities are particularly vulnerable, leading to vision problems, kidney damage, and nerve issues. This is why diabetes is often called a "silent killer"—the damage happens slowly over time, often without immediate symptoms.

The Role of Insulin in Regulating Blood Sugar

Insulin is a hormone that plays a critical role in controlling blood sugar levels. In a healthy body, insulin is released by the pancreas in response to rising blood sugar levels after you eat. It helps move glucose from the blood into the cells, where it's used as fuel. Think of insulin as a delivery driver, picking up glucose from the blood and dropping it off inside your cells, like a courier making deliveries to houses. In people with diabetes, this delivery system breaks down. Without insulin or with reduced insulin sensitivity, glucose stays in the bloodstream, leading to high blood sugar. Proper insulin management, whether through medication or lifestyle changes, is essential to keeping blood sugar levels in check and preventing long-term damage.

Short-Term Effects of Poor Glucose Control

If glucose is not managed effectively, diabetes can have both immediate and long-term effects. In the short term, poorly controlled blood sugar can lead to extreme highs (hyperglycemia) or lows (hypoglycemia). Hyperglycemia can cause symptoms such as excessive thirst, frequent urination, and fatigue. Imagine overloading a washing machine with too much water—it can't keep up and starts to overflow. This is how your body feels when your blood sugar levels are too high. On the other hand, hypoglycemia—low blood sugar—can cause dizziness, confusion, and even fainting. It's like running a car on an empty tank; eventually, it stalls. Maintaining balanced blood sugar levels is key to preventing these immediate dangers.

The Long-Term Consequences of Poor Blood Sugar Control

If high blood sugar is left unchecked for years, the long-term health consequences are serious. Cardiovascular disease is one of the leading causes of death for people with diabetes, as prolonged high blood sugar damages the heart and blood vessels. Diabetes also increases the risk of developing chronic kidney disease because the kidneys work overtime to filter excess glucose. Over time, this can lead to kidney failure. Imagine forcing a filter to process too much liquid day after day; eventually, it wears out. Nerve damage, or diabetic neuropathy, is another common outcome. This can cause pain, tingling, and even loss of feeling, particularly in the hands and feet. If left untreated, it can lead to infections and amputations. The risk of blindness also increases as high blood sugar damages the tiny blood vessels in the eyes, leading to diabetic retinopathy. This slow, cumulative damage underscores the importance of managing blood sugar effectively over the long term.

Diabetes and Its Impact on the Immune System

Diabetes doesn't just affect glucose regulation; it also impacts the immune system, making it harder for your body to fight off infections. Elevated blood sugar weakens white blood cells, which are critical for immune response. Think of your immune system as a security team protecting a building. When the team is compromised, intruders (infections) can easily slip in. People with diabetes are more susceptible to common infections like the flu or urinary tract infections, and these infections often take longer to heal. Maintaining good glucose control can help bolster your immune system and reduce the risk of complications from illnesses.

The Psychological Toll of Diabetes

Managing diabetes takes a significant mental and emotional toll on those affected. Constant monitoring of blood sugar levels, calculating insulin doses, and worrying about the long-term complications can lead to stress, anxiety, and even depression. It's like carrying a weight on your shoulders every day, with no break. The burden of managing diabetes can sometimes feel overwhelming, particularly for those who develop complications or face a higher risk of long-term health problems. Seeking support, whether through counseling, support groups, or simply talking with loved ones, can help ease the mental strain of managing this condition. It's important to understand that managing diabetes isn't just about physical health but mental well-being, too.

Preventing Long-Term Complications with Proper Management

While the potential long-term effects of diabetes are serious, they are not inevitable. With proper management, many of the complications associated with diabetes can be delayed or even prevented. Regular monitoring of blood sugar levels, maintaining a healthy diet, exercising, and taking medications as prescribed are critical to managing the condition. It's like maintaining a car—regular tune-ups, checking the oil, and addressing small issues before they become bigger problems are all ways to keep the car running smoothly for years. Similarly, staying on top of diabetes management helps keep your body functioning well and reduces the risk of long-term health issues. By keeping your blood sugar levels within a healthy range, you can significantly reduce the damage that high blood sugar causes over time.

Lifestyle Changes to Improve Glucose Management

Managing diabetes isn't just about medications—it's about making long-term lifestyle changes that support better glucose control. Simple habits like eating a balanced diet with plenty of fiber, getting regular physical activity, and staying hydrated can make a huge difference in managing blood sugar levels. Think of it as building a strong foundation for a house. Each healthy habit is like a brick, and together, they create a structure that supports your long-term health. These changes don't have to be dramatic, either. Small, sustainable steps—like switching to whole grains, taking a walk after meals, or drinking more water—can gradually improve your glucose control and help prevent complications   down   the   line.

The Role of Regular Checkups and Monitoring

Finally, regular checkups with your healthcare provider are an essential part of diabetes management. These visits are more than just routine—they are critical opportunities to catch any potential complications early and make necessary adjustments to your treatment plan. Think of your doctor as your personal mechanic for managing diabetes, checking under the hood, and making sure everything is running as it should. Regular blood tests, eye exams, and kidney function tests help track the progression of the disease and catch any signs of damage before they become severe. Staying proactive with your health is key to living a long and healthy life with diabetes.

Conclusion: Taking Control of Your Long-Term   Health

Diabetes is a lifelong condition, but it doesn't have to dictate your future. By understanding how it affects glucose and your body, and by taking active steps to manage your blood sugar, you can significantly reduce the risk of long-term complications. Maintaining a healthy lifestyle, regularly monitoring blood sugar levels, and staying in touch with your healthcare team are all essential tools for protecting your long-term health. With the right strategies, it's entirely possible to live a full, healthy life despite diabetes.

CHAPTER 8:

FOODS THAT IMPACT BLOOD SUGAR

How Diet Choices Can Raise or Lower Glucose Levels

Understanding the Link Between Food and Glucose Levels

What you eat directly impacts your glucose levels. When you consume food, especially carbohydrates, your body breaks it down into glucose, which enters your bloodstream. The speed at which glucose enters the bloodstream and how much enters depends on the type of food you eat. Imagine your body as a car, and glucose is the fuel. Some fuels (foods) burn quickly, sending energy (glucose) rushing through the system, while others release energy slowly, providing a steady, long-lasting source. Understanding which foods cause rapid spikes and which offer sustained energy is crucial for managing glucose levels effectively.

Carbohydrates: The Main Player in Glucose Control

Carbohydrates are often viewed as the primary culprit when it comes to elevated glucose levels. This is because they are the macronutrients most quickly converted into glucose. However, not all carbs are created equal. Simple carbohydrates, found in foods like white bread, sugary snacks, and soda, are rapidly broken down into glucose, leading to quick spikes in blood sugar levels. It's like throwing dry leaves onto a fire—instant flames, but they die down quickly, leaving you feeling tired and hungry again. On the other hand, complex carbohydrates, found in whole grains, vegetables, and legumes, take longer to digest. They act like logs on a fire, burning slowly and releasing glucose gradually, helping to maintain more stable blood sugar levels throughout the day.

The Glycemic Index: A Tool for Managing Glucose

A useful tool for understanding how different foods affect blood sugar is the glycemic index (GI). This system ranks foods based on how quickly they raise glucose levels after being consumed. Foods with a high GI, like white rice or pastries, cause a rapid rise in blood sugar, while low-GI foods, such as lentils or quinoa, result in a slower, more controlled release of glucose. Picture a roller coaster: high-GI foods send your blood sugar levels up rapidly, only to come crashing down shortly after. In contrast, low-GI foods offer a smooth, gradual ride with fewer ups and downs. Choosing low-GI foods can help keep blood sugar levels stable, reducing the risk of spikes and crashes that can leave you feeling sluggish or irritable.

Fiber: The Unsung Hero in Glucose Regulation

Fiber, found in fruits, vegetables, whole grains, and legumes, plays a key role in controlling glucose levels. Unlike other carbohydrates, fiber is not digested or absorbed by the body. Instead, it passes through the digestive system, helping to slow down the absorption of glucose. Think of fiber as a traffic cop, regulating the flow of glucose into your bloodstream, ensuring it enters slowly and steadily. By incorporating more high-fiber foods into your diet, you can prevent sharp increases in blood sugar. For example, pairing a high-fiber food like an apple with a protein-rich food like almond butter can further moderate glucose spikes, keeping your levels more balanced throughout the day.

The Role of Protein and Fat in Blood Sugar Stability

Protein and fats don't have a direct impact on blood sugar levels like carbohydrates do, but they play a critical role in managing glucose. When you eat a meal rich in protein or healthy fats, the digestion process slows down, which in turn slows the absorption of glucose. It's like adding a governor to the engine of your car, preventing it from going too fast too quickly. Foods like eggs, fish, nuts, and avocados not only provide essential nutrients but also help buffer the release of glucose into the bloodstream. Including them in your meals can help prevent the sharp rises in blood sugar that typically follow carbohydrate-heavy meals.

The Hidden Dangers of Processed Foods and Sugars

Processed foods, especially those high in added sugars, are some of the worst offenders when it comes to elevating glucose levels. These foods are often stripped of their fiber and other beneficial nutrients, making them easy to digest and rapidly absorbed into the bloodstream. Imagine pouring gasoline on a fire—it creates a burst of energy, but it's short-lived, leaving you craving more. Sugary drinks like sodas and energy drinks are especially dangerous because they cause glucose levels to spike almost immediately. Even seemingly "healthy" processed foods, like flavored yogurt or granola bars, can be loaded with hidden sugars. Always check labels for added sugars and opt for whole, unprocessed foods whenever possible to keep your glucose levels in check.

Meal Timing and Its Impact on Glucose Levels
What you eat is important, but when you eat can also affect glucose levels. Large meals, especially those high in carbohydrates, can cause significant spikes in blood sugar, while smaller, more frequent meals may help keep

glucose levels stable. It's similar to filling a balloon with air—if you add too much at once, it's more likely to burst. By eating smaller, balanced meals throughout the day, you prevent your blood sugar from spiking and crashing. Additionally, spacing out your meals evenly, rather than eating a large meal after hours of fasting, helps maintain more consistent glucose levels.

The Effect of Alcohol on Glucose Levels Alcohol is often overlooked when discussing diet and glucose levels, but it can have a significant impact. Alcohol initially lowers blood sugar, especially when consumed on an empty stomach, as it interferes with the liver's ability to release glucose into the bloodstream. However, after the initial drop, alcohol can cause a delayed spike in blood sugar, particularly if consumed in sugary cocktails or alongside carb-heavy foods. It's like pressing the brakes hard and then slamming the gas pedal—the sudden drop followed by a rise can throw your glucose levels out of balance. If you do choose to drink, it's best to do so in moderation and avoid sugary mixers to minimize the impact on your glucose levels.

Hydration and Its Role in Glucose Regulation
Drinking enough water is another simple yet effective way to help regulate glucose levels. When you're dehydrated, your body produces a hormone called vasopressin, which signals the kidneys to retain water. However, vasopressin also prompts the liver to release more glucose into the bloodstream. Picture a water dam holding back a reservoir. When the dam is low on water, the flow of glucose increases downstream, raising your blood sugar levels. Staying properly hydrated keeps this dam functioning smoothly and prevents unnecessary glucose release. Aim to drink water regularly throughout the day, especially before meals, to help manage glucose levels more effectively.

How Specific Diet Choices Affect Long-Term Health

The food choices you make daily don't just affect your glucose levels in the short term; they also influence your long-term health. Diets high in refined sugars, processed foods, and simple carbohydrates can lead to insulin resistance, increasing the risk of Type 2 diabetes. It's like wearing down the keys on a keyboard—eventually, they don't work as well. Over time, consistently elevated blood sugar levels can contribute to chronic conditions such as heart disease, stroke, and kidney failure. On the flip side, a diet rich in whole grains, lean proteins, healthy fats, and fiber can help reduce the risk of these complications, supporting better overall glucose control and long-term health.

Practical Tips for Balancing Glucose Levels Through Diet
Understanding the relationship between diet and glucose is one thing, but applying it to everyday life is another. Here are some practical tips to help keep your glucose levels stable:

- Combine Carbs with Protein and Fat: Instead of eating carbohydrates alone, pair them with a source of protein or healthy fat to slow down glucose absorption. For example, instead of plain toast, have it with avocado or nut butter.

- Opt for Whole Grains: Replace refined grains like white rice and white bread with whole grains like quinoa, oats, or whole wheat products. These foods digest more slowly and help maintain steady blood sugar levels.

- Limit Sugary Beverages: Water, herbal teas, or sparkling water with a slice of lemon are great alternatives to sugary drinks that can cause rapid glucose spikes.

- Increase Fiber Intake: Make a conscious effort to include more fiber-rich foods like vegetables, legumes, and whole fruits in your meals. Fiber helps regulate glucose by slowing down digestion.

- Watch Your Portions: Eating large portions, even of healthy foods, can lead to higher glucose levels. Be mindful of your portion sizes, especially with carbohydrate-rich meals.

Conclusion: Taking Control of Your Glucose Levels
Diet plays a fundamental role in regulating glucose levels, and making smart food choices can make a world of difference in your blood sugar management. By focusing on whole foods, balancing your macronutrients, and staying hydrated, you can effectively

control your glucose levels and support long-term health. Remember, managing glucose isn't about extreme diets or cutting out entire food groups; it's about making sustainable, balanced choices that nourish your body while keeping your blood sugar in check. Small, consistent changes to your diet can have a profound impact on your overall well-being and glucose management.

CHAPTER 9:

MONITORING YOUR BLOOD SUGAR

Effective Ways To Track And Understand Your Glucose Levels

The Importance of Monitoring Glucose Levels

Tracking your glucose levels is essential for maintaining overall health and preventing complications related to high or low blood sugar. Imagine driving a car without a speedometer; you wouldn't know when to slow down or speed up. Similarly, understanding your glucose levels helps you make informed dietary and lifestyle choices. By keeping an eye on how food, exercise, stress, and other factors impact your blood sugar, you can take control of your health and prevent the rollercoaster effects of glucose fluctuations. Monitoring your levels not only provides immediate feedback but also offers insights that can lead to long-term health improvements.

Choosing The Right Glucose Monitoring Method

There are several methods available for tracking glucose levels, each with its own advantages and disadvantages. The most common methods include traditional finger-prick blood glucose meters, continuous glucose monitors (CGMs), and laboratory testing.

- Finger-Prick Blood Glucose Meters: These portable devices require a small blood sample, typically from a finger prick. You can get results in seconds, making them great for immediate feedback. However, you need to remember to test regularly, and the process can be inconvenient for some. It's similar to using a compass; it gives you a quick direction but doesn't provide a full map.

- Continuous Glucose Monitors (CGMs): CGMs provide real-time glucose readings through a small sensor placed under the skin. This method allows you to see trends over time, making it easier to understand how different foods and activities affect your glucose levels. It's like having a GPS system in your car that shows your speed and direction continuously, helping you make adjustments on the fly.

- Laboratory Testing: Regular blood tests done by healthcare professionals can provide detailed insights into your glucose levels. This method is less convenient for day-to-day monitoring but can be beneficial for understanding long-term trends. Think of this as an annual check-up for your car—important but not something you do every day.

Establishing A Routine For Monitoring
Developing a consistent monitoring routine is crucial for effective glucose tracking. Determine when and how often you'll check your levels. For instance, if you are using a blood glucose meter, you might test before meals and a couple of hours after eating to see how your body responds to different foods. If you're using a CGM, you can set alerts for when your glucose levels go too high or low. It's like watering a garden—you need to check it regularly to know when it needs more water or less.

Creating a schedule helps you build a habit, and consistency is key. You might find it helpful to set reminders on your phone or keep a logbook to note your readings and the circumstances surrounding them, such as what you ate, your physical activity, and how you were feeling at the time. This data can help you recognize patterns, making it easier to manage your glucose levels effectively.

Understanding The Data: What Do Your Numbers Mean?

Once you have your glucose readings, it's essential to understand what they mean. Normal fasting glucose levels typically range from 70 to 100 mg/dL, while post-meal levels should ideally be below 180 mg/dL two hours after eating. However, individual targets can vary based on personal health conditions and goals.

If your readings consistently fall outside these ranges, it's time to investigate further. Elevated blood sugar may indicate that your body isn't using insulin effectively, while low blood sugar could be a sign that you need to adjust your diet or medication. This understanding is crucial for making informed decisions about your diet and lifestyle. Imagine your glucose numbers as signals from your body, guiding you toward healthier choices.

Using Apps And Technology To Aid Tracking

In today's digital age, there are many apps and devices designed to help you track and understand your glucose levels. These tools can simplify the process and provide additional insights. Many glucose meters now come with Bluetooth capabilities, allowing them to sync with your smartphone.

Apps like MySugr, Glucose Buddy, and Diabetes:M allow you to log your readings, meals, and activities in one place. Some even offer visualizations of your data, helping you identify trends over time. It's like using a fitness tracker for your glucose—providing you with real-time data and encouraging you to stay on track.

Moreover, some CGMs have dedicated apps that show your glucose levels in real-time, allowing you to see how your levels change throughout the day and night. You can use these tools to set alerts for high or low blood sugar, helping you respond promptly to changes.

Keeping A Food Diary For Better Insights
One of the most effective ways to understand your glucose levels is by keeping a food diary. By logging everything you eat, along with your corresponding glucose readings, you can identify patterns and triggers.

Start by noting down your meals and snacks, the ingredients used, and portion sizes. After eating, check your glucose levels and record the readings in your diary. Over time, you may notice that certain foods cause higher spikes than others, helping you make more informed dietary choices. For example, you might find that eating white bread leads to higher glucose levels than whole grain, prompting you to switch to healthier options.

This diary doesn't have to be complicated; a simple notebook or a notes app on your phone will suffice. The key is to be consistent and honest about what you consume. This exercise is akin to keeping a travel journal—you document your journey to gain insights that will inform your future decisions.

Learning From Trends: Adjusting Your Diet And Lifestyle

Once you've gathered enough data, take some time to analyze it. Look for trends in your readings and consider how your diet, exercise, stress levels, and sleep patterns may be influencing your glucose levels.

For example, if you notice that your glucose spikes significantly after eating a particular meal, consider adjusting your ingredients or portion sizes. You might also find that your glucose levels drop after exercising, prompting you to incorporate more physical activity into your routine. This reflective process is like reviewing a game tape—assessing what works and what doesn't, allowing you to strategize for future success.

If you consistently notice troubling patterns, it may be beneficial to consult with a healthcare professional. They can help you interpret your data and provide personalized advice on dietary and lifestyle changes that can help you manage your glucose levels effectively.

Engaging With Healthcare Providers: A Collaborative Approach
Regular consultations with healthcare professionals are vital for understanding your glucose management. Share your tracking data, including your food diary and any trends you've noticed, during your appointments.

This information can help your healthcare provider tailor their advice to your specific needs. They might suggest adjusting your medication, recommending dietary changes, or even referring you to a dietitian or nutritionist. This collaboration is key to successful glucose management; it's not just about tracking numbers but engaging in a two-way dialogue about your health. It's like having a coach to guide you through your health journey, providing support and expertise as you navigate your path.

Celebrating Progress and Setting Goals
Tracking glucose levels is not just about

identifying problems; it's also an opportunity to celebrate progress. Take the time to acknowledge your successes, whether it's maintaining stable glucose levels, sticking to your dietary goals, or improving your understanding of your body's signals.

Setting realistic, achievable goals can help keep you motivated. For example, aim to include more whole foods in your diet or exercise for a certain number of minutes each week. Celebrating small victories along the way, like trying a new healthy recipe or reaching a glucose target, reinforces positive behavior and keeps you on track.

Think of this process as a journey—enjoy the ride, learn from the bumps, and celebrate the milestones. The more engaged you are with tracking your glucose levels, the more empowered you'll feel in managing your health.

Conclusion: Taking Charge of Your Glucose Health
Effective tracking and understanding of glucose levels are crucial for maintaining good

health, particularly for those managing conditions like diabetes. By choosing the right monitoring methods, establishing a routine, utilizing technology, and engaging with healthcare providers, you can gain valuable insights into your body and make informed decisions about your diet and lifestyle.

With consistent effort and dedication, tracking your glucose levels can transform from a daunting task into a valuable tool for achieving better health. Embrace the journey, learn from your experiences, and take charge of your glucose health—after all, knowledge is power when it comes to living a balanced and healthy life.

CHAPTER 10:

EXERCISE AND GLUCOSE CONTROL

The Role of Physical Activity in Stabilizing Blood Sugar

Understanding Blood Sugar Levels
Blood sugar, or glucose, is our body's main source of energy. Just as a car needs fuel to run smoothly, our bodies require glucose to function properly. However, not all fuel is created equal. When blood sugar levels fluctuate too much—whether spiking too high or dropping too low—it can lead to various health issues, particularly for those with conditions like diabetes. Imagine driving a car with inconsistent fuel supply; it would stall and sputter, making the journey unpredictable. Similarly, maintaining stable blood sugar levels is crucial for a smooth ride through life.

How Physical Activity Affects Blood Sugar
Physical activity is one of the most effective tools for stabilizing blood sugar levels. When you engage in exercise, your muscles require

energy, and they draw on glucose for that energy. This process lowers the amount of glucose in your bloodstream. For instance, when you go for a brisk walk or engage in a sport, your muscles use glucose as fuel, effectively reducing blood sugar levels.

Additionally, regular physical activity increases insulin sensitivity, meaning your body's cells are more effective at using insulin to absorb glucose. Think of insulin as a key that opens the door to your cells, allowing glucose to enter. With increased insulin sensitivity, that door opens more easily, allowing for smoother energy usage. This is akin to oiling the hinges of a door—it makes opening it much easier.

Types of Physical Activity and Their Benefits

Different types of physical activity can have unique effects on blood sugar levels. Broadly, these activities can be categorized into aerobic exercise, strength training, and flexibility exercises.

- Aerobic Exercise: This includes activities like walking, running, cycling, or swimming.

Aerobic exercise is fantastic for immediately lowering blood sugar levels as it helps your body use glucose efficiently. For example, if you take a 30-minute brisk walk after a meal, you may notice a decrease in your blood sugar levels, as your muscles actively draw on the glucose consumed.

- Strength Training: Lifting weights or doing resistance exercises builds muscle mass, which is essential for glucose metabolism. More muscle means your body has a larger reservoir to draw glucose from, helping stabilize blood sugar levels over time. Imagine a sponge soaking up water; more sponge (muscle) means more water (glucose) can be absorbed. Incorporating strength training into your routine, even twice a week, can significantly impact your long-term glucose management.

- Flexibility Exercises: Activities like yoga and stretching may not directly lower blood sugar levels, but they contribute to overall physical activity and improve mental well-being. Managing stress through these exercises can prevent stress-related blood sugar spikes.

Think of flexibility exercises as maintenance for your body; they keep everything running smoothly and prevent injuries, making it easier to stay active.

Establishing A Regular Exercise Routine
To reap the benefits of physical activity on blood sugar levels, consistency is key. Establishing a regular exercise routine can help create lasting habits. Aim for at least 150 minutes of moderate-intensity aerobic activity each week, combined with two or more days of strength training.

Start small; if the idea of 150 minutes feels daunting, break it down into manageable chunks. For instance, commit to 10-minute walks throughout the day. Gradually increase the duration and intensity as you become more comfortable. Consistency is like watering a plant; it nurtures growth over time, leading to healthier habits and better blood sugar management.

Listening to Your Body: Timing Matters
The timing of physical activity can significantly impact blood sugar levels. Engaging in

exercise at strategic times can amplify its benefits. For example, doing light aerobic activity after meals can help control post-meal blood sugar spikes.

If you notice your blood sugar levels tend to rise after eating, consider going for a short walk. This simple change can serve as a natural remedy, helping your body manage glucose levels more effectively. Just like adjusting the thermostat can create a more comfortable environment in your home, adjusting the timing of your exercise can lead to better blood sugar control.

The Importance of Hydration and Nutrition
Hydration and nutrition play a crucial role in how physical activity affects blood sugar. When you're properly hydrated, your body can function optimally, which enhances your performance during exercise. Aim to drink water before, during, and after your workouts. Think of hydration as oil in an engine; without it, everything can get gummed up and function poorly.

Nutrition is equally important. Fueling your body with the right foods before and after exercise can help stabilize blood sugar levels. For instance, a balanced meal containing complex carbohydrates, protein, and healthy fats can provide sustained energy, while snacks like nuts or yogurt can offer a quick boost if you feel your energy dip. Eating well is like putting high-quality fuel in your car; it allows for better performance and longevity.

Understanding How Different Activities Affect Blood Sugar
Every individual responds differently to various types of physical activity. It's essential to pay attention to how your body reacts to different workouts. After engaging in aerobic exercise, you might notice a quick drop in blood sugar, while strength training may result in a more gradual effect. Keeping a journal to track your workouts and corresponding blood sugar levels can provide valuable insights.

For example, if you go for a run and see a significant drop in your blood sugar, you might want to have a small snack before your run next time. Conversely, if you find that strength training causes minimal fluctuations in your blood sugar, you may decide to incorporate it more frequently into your routine. This personalized approach is like fine-tuning a musical instrument; small adjustments can lead to a much better performance.

Incorporating Movement into Daily Life
Physical activity doesn't have to be limited to structured workouts. Incorporating more movement into your daily routine can be just as beneficial for blood sugar stabilization. Simple changes, such as taking the stairs instead of the elevator, parking farther from your destination, or doing household chores, can add up over time.

Think of these small activities as deposits in a savings account; over time, they accumulate and lead to substantial benefits for your health. Setting reminders to move, such as standing up every hour or doing short bursts of activity throughout the day, can help create a more active lifestyle.

Overcoming Barriers to Physical Activity
Many people encounter barriers that can

make regular physical activity challenging. Common obstacles include time constraints, lack of motivation, or physical limitations. However, overcoming these barriers is possible with a few strategies.

First, consider your schedule; even short bursts of activity can be effective. Try setting aside just 10-15 minutes in your day to engage in something you enjoy, whether it's dancing, gardening, or playing with your kids. Finding activities that you genuinely enjoy will keep you motivated.

If physical limitations are a concern, consult with a healthcare provider or a fitness expert to design a safe and effective exercise plan tailored to your needs. Just as you would ask for directions when lost, seeking guidance can lead you to the best route for achieving your goals.

Building a Support System
Having a support system can make a world of difference when it comes to maintaining a physical activity routine. Engaging with friends, family, or support groups can provide

encouragement and accountability.

Consider finding a workout buddy or joining a class in your community. This not only makes exercise more enjoyable but also fosters a sense of belonging. Sharing your goals with others can motivate you to stick to your routine, just as having a travel companion makes the journey more enjoyable and memorable.

Celebrating Progress

Finally, don't forget to celebrate your achievements along the way. Acknowledging your progress, whether it's completing a workout, hitting a blood sugar target, or simply sticking to your routine, reinforces positive behaviors.

Set small, achievable goals and reward yourself when you reach them. This could be as simple as treating yourself to a movie night or buying new workout gear. Recognizing your accomplishments is essential for sustaining motivation and commitment. Just like celebrating a birthday brings joy and excitement, celebrating your health milestones fosters a positive mindset.

Conclusion: Taking Charge of Your Blood Sugar Through Physical Activity
Physical activity plays a vital role in stabilizing blood sugar levels and promoting overall health. By understanding how different types of exercise affect your body, establishing a regular routine, and incorporating movement into your daily life, you can take charge of your glucose management. Remember to stay hydrated, fuel your body with nutritious foods, and listen to your body's signals.

With consistency, determination, and the support of others, you can create a sustainable lifestyle that enhances your well-being and empowers you to live life to the fullest. Embrace the journey, celebrate your successes, and keep moving toward your health goals—your body will thank you for it!

CHAPTER 11:

STRESS AND BLOOD SUGAR FLUCTUATIONS

Why Stress Management Is Key for Healthy Glucose Levels

Understanding the Connection Between Stress and Blood Sugar Stress is an inevitable part of life, but how we respond to it can have significant effects on our health, particularly when it comes to blood sugar levels. When faced with stress, our bodies enter a state known as "fight or flight." This physiological response releases hormones like adrenaline and cortisol, which prepare us to react quickly to perceived threats. While this response was beneficial for our ancestors, modern stressors—like work deadlines or financial worries—can lead to prolonged exposure to these hormones, which can wreak havoc on our blood sugar levels. Imagine driving a car with the gas pedal constantly pressed; it can lead to overheating and engine failure over time. Similarly, chronic stress keeps our bodies in a constant state of readiness, leading to elevated blood sugar levels and other health issues.

The Impact of Stress Hormones on Blood Sugar

When cortisol is released, it prompts the liver to release glucose into the bloodstream for quick energy. While this response is helpful in short bursts, frequent spikes in blood sugar due to stress can lead to insulin resistance over time. This means that your body's cells become less responsive to insulin, making it harder for glucose to enter the cells and leading to elevated blood sugar levels. Consider this analogy: if you constantly knock on a door but no one answers, you'll eventually stop knocking. In the same way, your cells begin to ignore insulin when it's consistently present in high amounts due to stress, which can lead to chronic blood sugar issues.

Recognizing Stress Symptoms

Recognizing the signs of stress is the first step in managing it effectively. Symptoms can manifest physically, emotionally, and behaviorally. Physical signs might include headaches, fatigue, muscle tension, or digestive issues. Emotionally, you may feel anxious, irritable, or overwhelmed. Behaviorally, stress might lead to changes in eating habits, such as overeating or not eating at all, which can further impact glucose levels. Imagine your body as a complex machine; when one part isn't functioning well, it affects the whole system. Being aware of these signs allows you to take proactive steps to manage your stress before it impacts your health.

The Role of Mindfulness in Stress Reduction

Mindfulness practices, such as meditation and deep-breathing exercises, can be incredibly effective in managing stress and, by extension, stabilizing blood sugar levels. Mindfulness encourages you to focus on the present moment and observe your thoughts and feelings without judgment. For example, when feeling stressed about an upcoming meeting, take a moment to breathe deeply and bring your attention to the here and now. Picture a balloon; as you inhale, imagine it inflating, and as you exhale, visualize it deflating. This simple exercise can help calm your mind and reduce stress. Research has shown that practicing mindfulness can lower cortisol levels, ultimately supporting healthier blood sugar levels.

Exercise: A Powerful Stress Reliever
Regular physical activity is one of the most effective ways to manage stress. Exercise releases endorphins, the body's natural feel-good hormones, which help improve mood and reduce anxiety. Whether it's a brisk walk, a dance class, or lifting weights, moving your body can serve as a powerful outlet for stress. Imagine stress as a soda can; when shaken, it builds pressure. Exercise is like opening the can and releasing that pressure. Not only does it alleviate stress, but it also helps improve insulin sensitivity and glucose metabolism, creating a win-win situation for your health. Aim for at least 150 minutes of moderate-intensity exercise each week to reap these benefits.

Nutrition's Role in Stress Management
What you eat also plays a critical role in how your body manages stress and blood sugar levels. Stress can lead to unhealthy eating

habits, such as seeking comfort foods that are high in sugar and unhealthy fats. These foods can cause rapid spikes in blood sugar, creating a vicious cycle of stress and unhealthy eating. Instead, focus on a balanced diet rich in whole foods, such as fruits, vegetables, whole grains, lean proteins, and healthy fats. Think of your body as a garden; nourishing it with wholesome foods fosters growth and resilience. Foods rich in magnesium, omega-3 fatty acids, and antioxidants can help combat stress and stabilize blood sugar levels.

Sleep: The Overlooked Component of Stress Management

Adequate sleep is often overlooked when discussing stress management, but it plays a vital role in regulating blood sugar. Lack of sleep can lead to increased cortisol levels and decreased insulin sensitivity, making it harder for your body to manage glucose levels. Imagine a phone running low on battery; it can't function properly until recharged. Similarly, your body needs sufficient rest to recharge and perform optimally. Aim for 7-9 hours of quality sleep each night. Establish a relaxing bedtime routine, such as reading or gentle stretching, to signal to your body that it's time to wind down.

Building a Support System
Having a strong support system can significantly help in managing stress. Whether it's friends, family, or a professional counselor, talking about your stressors can provide relief and new perspectives. Share your feelings and experiences with trusted individuals who can offer encouragement and understanding. Picture a safety net; when you fall, it catches you and prevents further harm. A supportive community acts similarly, providing the necessary support to help you navigate life's challenges. Joining a support group, whether in-person or online, can also foster a sense of belonging and shared understanding, making it easier to cope with stressors.

Creating a Personal Stress Management Plan
Creating a personalized stress management plan can empower you to take control of your stress and blood sugar levels. Start by identifying your stress triggers and

determining effective coping strategies for each. Consider incorporating a mix of mindfulness practices, exercise, healthy eating, and social support into your routine. Make a list of activities that help you relax, whether it's listening to music, taking a bath, or engaging in a hobby. Keep this list handy, so when stress arises, you have ready-to-go strategies at your fingertips. Think of it as packing a survival kit; when faced with a challenge, you can rely on your toolkit to navigate through.

Regular Monitoring of Blood Sugar Levels
If you have a condition like diabetes, regular monitoring of your blood sugar levels is essential for managing stress effectively. Keeping track of how your blood sugar responds to different stressors can provide valuable insights. For instance, you might notice that a stressful meeting causes your levels to spike, prompting you to employ stress-reduction techniques before the next one. Think of it as a GPS system guiding you on your health journey; knowing your current location (blood sugar levels) helps you adjust your route (stress management strategies)

accordingly.

Seeking Professional Help When Necessary

Sometimes, stress can become overwhelming, and seeking professional help is a sign of strength, not weakness. A mental health professional can provide you with tools and techniques to manage stress effectively. Therapy can help you uncover underlying issues contributing to your stress and develop healthier coping strategies. Just as you'd consult a mechanic for car troubles, seeking help from a professional ensures you receive the best care for your mental health.

Conclusion: Prioritizing Stress Management for Better Health

Stress management is not just a luxury; it's a necessity for maintaining healthy glucose levels and overall well-being. By understanding the connection between stress and blood sugar, recognizing stress symptoms, and implementing effective coping strategies, you can take control of your health. Incorporate mindfulness practices, regular exercise, nutritious eating, adequate sleep, and a supportive community into your life.

Monitor your blood sugar levels and don't hesitate to seek professional help when needed. By prioritizing stress management, you are investing in a healthier future for yourself. Just as a well-tended garden flourishes, so too will your health when nurtured with care and attention. Embrace the journey toward better stress management, and in turn, create a path to healthier glucose levels and a more fulfilling life.

CHAPTER 12:

MEDICATIONS THAT INFLUENCE GLUCOSE

How Prescription Drugs Can Impact Your Blood Sugar Control

Understanding Prescription Drugs and Blood Sugar

Prescription medications play a crucial role in managing various health conditions, but they can also significantly influence blood sugar levels, particularly for individuals with diabetes or those at risk of developing it. Just like fuel can either power or hinder a vehicle, medications can have varying effects on your body's ability to regulate glucose. Understanding how specific drugs impact blood sugar can empower you to make informed decisions about your treatment options. This knowledge is vital, especially if you are managing diabetes or prediabetes.

Types of Medications That Affect Blood Sugar

Different classes of medications can affect

blood sugar in distinct ways. Some can raise blood sugar levels, while others may lower them. For instance, corticosteroids, commonly prescribed for inflammatory conditions like arthritis or asthma, can increase blood sugar levels by promoting gluconeogenesis, the process by which the liver produces glucose. Imagine your liver as a factory; when stressed, it works overtime to produce more products (glucose), potentially leading to a surplus that the body can't handle. On the other hand, certain medications like metformin are designed to improve insulin sensitivity, helping to lower blood sugar levels. Understanding the role of these medications is essential in managing your overall health.

Corticosteroids: The Sugar-Raising Culprits

Corticosteroids, such as prednisone, are powerful anti-inflammatory medications that can lead to elevated blood sugar levels. They can cause the body to become more insulin-resistant, meaning that the insulin produced is less effective at allowing glucose to enter the cells. For someone with diabetes, this can result in higher blood glucose readings. Think of it as a clogged sink; even though water (glucose) is flowing, it can't drain properly due to a blockage (insulin resistance). If you are prescribed corticosteroids, it's crucial to monitor your blood sugar closely, as these medications can significantly alter your usual readings.

Antipsychotics and Their Impact on Glucose Levels
Certain antipsychotic medications, particularly atypical antipsychotics, have also been linked to weight gain and insulin resistance, which can elevate blood sugar levels. Medications like olanzapine and clozapine are known to increase appetite and lead to metabolic changes. Picture your metabolism as a campfire; when it's stoked, it burns brightly, but when it's smothered, it burns out. These medications can smother your metabolism, leading to weight gain and making blood sugar management more challenging. If you are taking these medications, discuss with your healthcare provider about the potential effects on your blood sugar and explore strategies to mitigate them.

The Role of Diuretics in Blood Sugar Control

Diuretics, commonly prescribed to manage high blood pressure, can also influence blood sugar levels. Thiazide diuretics, in particular, may lead to an increase in blood sugar by decreasing insulin sensitivity. Consider this: if your body's cells are like tiny doors that open to let glucose in, diuretics can make those doors stick, preventing glucose from entering effectively. If you're on diuretics, monitor your blood sugar regularly and communicate with your healthcare provider about any changes you notice.

Beta-Blockers: The Double-Edged Sword

Beta-blockers, often used to treat hypertension and anxiety, can have mixed effects on blood sugar control. While they may not significantly raise blood sugar levels, they can mask the symptoms of low blood sugar (hypoglycemia). Imagine you're a firefighter; when the alarm goes off, you respond quickly to put out the fire. However, if the alarm malfunctions and doesn't sound when there's a fire (hypoglycemia), you could be caught off guard. This is particularly concerning for individuals with diabetes who may rely on these symptoms to manage their condition. It's essential to work closely with your healthcare provider if you're prescribed beta-blockers to ensure proper monitoring of your blood sugar levels.

Statins and Their Influence on Blood Sugar
Statins, which are prescribed to lower cholesterol, have been associated with slightly elevated blood sugar levels in some studies. While the increase may be modest, it's important to remain aware of how these medications may impact your glucose control, especially if you have other risk factors for diabetes. Think of it as balancing a scale; while statins help reduce cholesterol, they can add a little weight to the blood sugar side. If you're on statins, keep an open dialogue with your healthcare provider about how to monitor and manage any potential blood sugar changes.

Communication with Your Healthcare Provider
Open communication with your healthcare provider is vital when it comes to managing

blood sugar levels, especially if you're taking multiple medications. Keeping a detailed log of your blood sugar readings, medication schedule, and any side effects can provide valuable insights for your healthcare team. Think of this log as a roadmap; it helps both you and your provider navigate your treatment journey. By sharing this information, you can collaboratively adjust your treatment plan to better manage your blood sugar levels.

Lifestyle Modifications: A Complementary Approach

In addition to medication management, lifestyle modifications can play a crucial role in stabilizing blood sugar levels. Incorporating regular physical activity, a balanced diet rich in whole foods, and effective stress management techniques can enhance the effects of your medications. Imagine building a house; medications provide the foundation, but lifestyle changes are like the walls and roof that keep everything secure. Engaging in regular exercise can improve insulin sensitivity, making it easier for your body to utilize glucose effectively. Aim for at least 150 minutes of moderate-intensity exercise each week to support your blood sugar management.

Monitoring Blood Sugar Levels: A Proactive Approach

Regularly monitoring your blood sugar levels is essential for understanding how your body responds to medications and lifestyle changes. Use a continuous glucose monitor (CGM) or traditional glucose meter to track your levels and identify patterns. For instance, you might notice that certain medications lead to spikes in your blood sugar after meals. By recognizing these patterns, you can make informed decisions about your diet and medication regimen. Think of monitoring as a lighthouse guiding you through rocky waters; it helps you stay on course and avoid potential hazards.

Seeking Alternative Medications

If you experience significant blood sugar fluctuations due to prescription drugs, discuss alternative medications with your healthcare provider. There may be options that better suit your individual needs without adversely affecting your blood sugar levels. For example, if corticosteroids are necessary, your provider may recommend a lower dose or a shorter treatment duration. It's essential to approach this conversation openly and collaboratively, as finding the right balance between managing your primary health condition and maintaining stable blood sugar levels is crucial.

The Importance of Education and Empowerment

Education is a powerful tool in managing your health. By understanding how various medications impact blood sugar, you can take an active role in your treatment plan. Consider attending diabetes education classes or support groups to learn more about managing your condition effectively. Knowledge empowers you to advocate for your health and make informed decisions about your medications and lifestyle. Picture yourself as the captain of your health ship; the more you know, the better you can navigate the waters of prescription medications and blood sugar control.

Conclusion: Taking Charge of Your Blood Sugar

Prescription drugs can significantly impact blood sugar control, making it essential for individuals managing diabetes or prediabetes to stay informed. By understanding how different medications affect glucose levels, you can work collaboratively with your healthcare provider to optimize your treatment plan. Regular monitoring, open communication, and lifestyle modifications are critical components of effective blood sugar management.

Remember, you are not alone on this journey; a supportive healthcare team is there to guide you. With the right tools and knowledge, you can take charge of your health and make choices that promote stable blood sugar levels and overall well-being. Empower yourself through education, advocacy, and proactive management, and embark on a path toward better health.

CHAPTER 13:

NATURAL APPROACHES TO GLUCOSE MANAGEMENT

Alternative Ways to Maintain Stable Blood Sugar Levels

Introduction: Rethinking Blood Sugar Management

Maintaining stable blood sugar levels is essential for overall health, especially for those managing diabetes or prediabetes. While medications are a common approach, there are many alternative ways to naturally support blood sugar control. These methods often complement traditional treatments and can make a significant difference in how your body manages glucose. Think of your body as a finely tuned instrument—when everything works in harmony, it performs optimally. In this section, we'll explore several powerful strategies that go beyond conventional methods to help you maintain stable blood sugar levels effectively.

The Power of Balanced Nutrition
One of the most effective ways to stabilize blood sugar is through a well-balanced diet. The food you eat can either cause spikes in glucose or help keep it steady. Rather than focusing solely on eliminating carbohydrates, think of your diet as an opportunity to nourish your body with the right combinations of nutrients. Aim to balance complex carbohydrates, healthy fats, and lean proteins at each meal.

For example, instead of a plain bowl of oatmeal, which could raise blood sugar quickly, add some almond butter and chia seeds. These healthy fats and fibers slow down the absorption of glucose into the bloodstream, helping to prevent sharp spikes. Just like a steady stream of water fills a glass without overflowing, balancing macronutrients helps glucose enter your system slowly and steadily.

The Role of Fiber in Blood Sugar Control
Fiber is a game changer when it comes to managing blood sugar levels. Soluble fiber, found in foods like beans, oats, and flaxseeds,

acts like a sponge in your digestive system, slowing down the absorption of sugar and preventing those sudden glucose highs and lows. Picture a sponge soaking up water—it controls how fast the water spreads. In the same way, fiber controls how quickly sugar enters your bloodstream, offering a more stable energy flow throughout the day.

Incorporating high-fiber foods into your meals not only helps with blood sugar but also keeps you feeling full longer, reducing overeating and unnecessary snacking, which can contribute to glucose fluctuations. A simple tip is to swap out refined grains like white bread or pasta for whole grains like quinoa or barley, adding natural sources of fiber into your diet.

Hydration: An Underrated Strategy
Staying properly hydrated is often overlooked as a method to control blood sugar, but it plays a crucial role. Water helps flush excess sugar out of the bloodstream and supports overall metabolic function. Dehydration can lead to higher blood sugar levels because the concentration of glucose in the blood becomes more dense. Imagine trying to

dissolve sugar in a tiny amount of water—there's simply not enough liquid to dilute it properly. The same thing happens in your body when you're dehydrated.

To stay hydrated, focus on drinking water consistently throughout the day. Try adding a slice of lemon or cucumber for flavor, which can make it more enjoyable. Keep a water bottle nearby and sip frequently to avoid long periods without fluid intake. While sugary drinks and sodas should be avoided, herbal teas or sparkling water are great alternatives to plain water and can still keep your hydration levels in check.

Stress Reduction: A Key to Stabilizing Blood Sugar

Stress is an invisible but powerful driver of blood sugar fluctuations. When you're stressed, your body releases cortisol, a hormone that raises blood sugar to provide you with the energy needed for the "fight or flight" response. While this might be useful in emergencies, chronic stress can lead to consistently elevated glucose levels.

Mindfulness practices such as meditation, yoga, or deep breathing exercises can help reduce stress and lower cortisol levels, indirectly supporting better blood sugar control. Imagine stress as a pot of boiling water; mindfulness techniques act like removing the pot from the heat, allowing it to simmer down. Taking just five minutes each day for deep breathing can have a profound effect on your stress levels and, as a result, on your glucose stability.

Regular Movement: Small Changes, Big Impact

You don't need to run marathons to experience the blood sugar benefits of exercise. Simple, consistent movement throughout the day can significantly improve how your body handles glucose. Engaging in light physical activity after meals, such as a 10-15 minute walk, can help reduce blood sugar spikes by stimulating your muscles to use glucose more efficiently. Think of your muscles like a sponge that absorbs excess sugar when activated. By walking or doing gentle exercises, you can keep that sponge working all day.

Incorporating strength training exercises like lifting weights or using resistance bands a few times a week can also improve insulin sensitivity. This makes it easier for your body to utilize glucose without needing excessive amounts of insulin.

Even everyday activities such as cleaning, gardening, or taking the stairs can positively impact your blood sugar management. The key is consistency—small, regular movement adds up and helps keep your glucose levels in check.

Sleep: The Unsung Hero of Glucose Control

Quality sleep is often overlooked but plays a vital role in maintaining stable blood sugar levels. When you don't get enough rest, your body's ability to regulate insulin is compromised, leading to higher blood sugar levels the next day. Think of sleep as the time when your body recharges its batteries. Just like a phone that functions poorly on low battery, your body struggles to manage glucose when it's sleep-deprived.

Aim for 7-9 hours of sleep per night, and establish a relaxing bedtime routine to help you unwind. This might include reading, meditating, or practicing deep breathing exercises. Avoiding screens before bed and limiting caffeine intake in the afternoon can also contribute to better sleep quality. Prioritizing rest allows your body to recover, making it easier to maintain steady blood sugar levels throughout the day.

Incorporating Probiotics for Better Gut Health

Your gut health has a direct influence on your blood sugar levels, and incorporating probiotics can support this connection. Probiotics are beneficial bacteria that help balance your gut microbiome, which plays a crucial role in digestion and overall metabolic health. Research suggests that an imbalanced gut can lead to insulin resistance and blood sugar fluctuations. Think of your gut as a garden—when it's well-maintained with healthy bacteria, everything grows and functions smoothly.

Foods rich in probiotics, such as yogurt, kefir, sauerkraut, and kimchi, can support your gut health and, in turn, improve your body's ability to regulate blood sugar. You can also consider taking probiotic supplements if dietary changes are difficult. Pairing probiotics with prebiotic foods like garlic, onions, and bananas provides the ideal environment for healthy bacteria to thrive, further promoting glucose stability.

The Power of Herbal Remedies
Certain herbs have long been used in traditional medicine to help regulate blood sugar levels. Cinnamon, for example, has been shown to improve insulin sensitivity and lower fasting blood sugar levels. Think of cinnamon as a natural "reset" button for your body's insulin response. It helps your cells recognize insulin more efficiently, making it easier for them to absorb glucose.

Other herbs like fenugreek and bitter melon have similar effects, promoting better glucose control. Incorporating these herbs into your diet can be as simple as adding cinnamon to your morning coffee or tea or cooking with fenugreek seeds. Always consult with your healthcare provider before using herbal supplements, especially if you're already taking medications for blood sugar management, to ensure there are no interactions.

The Importance of Mindful Eating
Mindful eating is a practice that encourages you to be fully present during meals, paying attention to hunger and fullness cues and savoring each bite. This approach can help prevent overeating and support more stable blood sugar levels. Imagine eating in slow motion—when you chew slowly and focus on your meal, your body has time to signal when it's full, reducing the likelihood of consuming excess calories that can lead to blood sugar spikes.

To practice mindful eating, eliminate distractions such as TV or your phone during meals. Focus on the taste, texture, and smell of your food, and take the time to enjoy it. Eating slowly allows your body to process the food more efficiently and can prevent large fluctuations in blood sugar levels that often occur after rushed meals.

Combining Strategies for Maximum Benefit

No single method will guarantee perfect blood sugar control, but combining multiple strategies can create a powerful synergy. By adopting a balanced diet, staying hydrated, managing stress, incorporating movement, prioritizing sleep, and exploring probiotics and herbal remedies, you can maintain more stable blood sugar levels naturally. Think of these methods as pieces of a puzzle—when they come together, they form a complete picture of optimal glucose management.

Consistency is key, and small changes made over time can lead to significant improvements in how your body regulates blood sugar. By understanding the various factors that influence glucose levels and taking proactive steps, you can better manage your health and prevent complications down the line.

Conclusion: Taking Charge of Your Blood Sugar

Maintaining stable blood sugar levels doesn't have to rely solely on medication. By incorporating these alternative methods, you can create a holistic approach to glucose management that supports your overall well-being. Whether through mindful eating, regular movement, or exploring the benefits of probiotics and herbs, there are plenty of ways to keep your blood sugar in check.

Ultimately, it's about finding the right balance for your body and lifestyle. With these strategies, you have the tools to take control of your health and enjoy greater stability in your blood sugar levels, contributing to a healthier and more vibrant life.

CHAPTER 14:

LONG-TERM STRATEGIES FOR GLUCOSE HEALTH

Creating Sustainable Habits for Lifelong Blood Sugar Balance

The Power of Consistent Habits
When it comes to maintaining balanced blood sugar levels over a lifetime, consistency is key. Developing sustainable habits is not just about short-term solutions but creating daily practices that become second nature. Think of these habits like building a house—you need a strong foundation to ensure it stands firm over time. In this case, your foundation is built on habits that support your blood sugar balance. The more consistent you are, the easier it becomes to manage your glucose levels and protect your long-term health.

Start Small and Build Gradually
One of the biggest mistakes people make when trying to improve their health is attempting to overhaul everything at once. This can lead to burnout and failure to stick

with new behaviors. Instead, the most effective way to create lasting habits is to start small and build gradually. Imagine trying to lift a heavy weight without training your muscles first—it's overwhelming and likely to result in injury. Similarly, changing too many aspects of your diet or lifestyle at once can feel exhausting.

For instance, if you're trying to eat healthier for better blood sugar control, begin by making one small adjustment, such as swapping sugary snacks for a piece of fruit or a handful of nuts. Once this becomes a habit, move on to the next change. By adding small habits one at a time, you allow them to become automatic, creating a snowball effect that leads to significant long-term improvement in glucose management.

Understand Your Personal Blood Sugar Triggers

Personalization is essential in creating sustainable habits, especially when it comes to blood sugar balance. Everyone's body responds differently to various foods, stress, and physical activity. Understanding your unique blood sugar triggers helps you develop habits tailored to your needs. Imagine each person's blood sugar regulation like a fingerprint—unique and highly individual.

One practical way to discover your triggers is by using a blood glucose monitor or a continuous glucose monitor (CGM) to track your responses to different meals, activities, or even stressors. Over time, patterns will emerge, and you can identify which foods cause spikes or which situations lead to blood sugar imbalances. Once you have this data, it becomes much easier to create habits that work specifically for you, making it more likely that you'll stick with them long term.

Design Your Environment for Success
Your environment has a powerful influence on your habits, and designing it in a way that supports blood sugar balance can make healthy choices more automatic. Think of your environment as a path that guides your behavior. If the path is full of obstacles, it's harder to stay on track. But if the path is clear, making the right choice becomes almost effortless.

Start by stocking your kitchen with nutrient-dense, low-glycemic foods that promote stable blood sugar. Keep high-sugar and highly processed foods out of sight, or better yet, out of the house entirely. If healthy foods like fresh vegetables, lean proteins, and healthy fats are readily available, you're more likely to reach for them when hunger strikes.

In the same way, design your daily routine to include opportunities for physical activity and stress management. Set up a dedicated space in your home for stretching or yoga, or keep a pair of walking shoes by the door to remind you to take a brisk walk. By creating an environment that supports blood sugar-friendly habits, you reduce the friction of making good choices.

Practice Mindful Eating to Stabilize Blood Sugar

Mindful eating is one of the most powerful tools for sustaining long-term blood sugar balance. It's not just about what you eat but how you eat. When you're distracted, rushed, or stressed during meals, you're more likely to overeat or make poor food choices, both of which can cause glucose spikes.

Mindful eating encourages you to slow down and fully experience your meals. Picture eating as a conversation between you and your body—if you're not paying attention, you miss the signals telling you when you're satisfied. To practice mindful eating, start by eliminating distractions during meals. Put away your phone, turn off the TV, and focus on the flavors, textures, and sensations of each bite. This helps you better recognize when you're full and prevents overeating, which can lead to blood sugar imbalances.

In addition, mindful eating involves being aware of the emotional drivers behind your food choices. Are you reaching for that sugary snack because you're truly hungry, or because you're stressed or bored? By becoming aware of these emotional triggers, you can develop healthier coping strategies that don't involve food, reducing unnecessary glucose spikes.

Incorporate Movement into Your Daily Routine

Regular physical activity is essential for managing blood sugar, but it doesn't mean you need to spend hours in the gym. The key to sustainability is incorporating movement into your daily routine in a way that feels enjoyable and natural. Think of exercise as a tool to "burn off" excess sugar and improve insulin sensitivity, much like adjusting the thermostat to control the temperature in your home.

You can start by adding simple movements throughout your day, such as walking, stretching, or even doing household chores. A brisk 10-minute walk after meals can help reduce blood sugar spikes, and it's a manageable activity that doesn't require a huge time commitment. The more you move, the more glucose your muscles use, which can prevent excess sugar from circulating in your bloodstream.

To make movement a sustainable habit, find activities you genuinely enjoy. Whether it's dancing, swimming, or hiking, doing something you love ensures you'll stick with it long term. Additionally, incorporating variety into your routine prevents boredom and helps keep your body engaged in different ways.

Develop a Stress-Management Routine
Stress has a significant impact on blood sugar levels. When you're stressed, your body releases cortisol, a hormone that raises blood sugar to provide energy for the "fight or flight" response. Chronic stress leads to consistently elevated blood sugar, making it more difficult to maintain balance.

The key to sustainable blood sugar management is developing habits that help you manage stress effectively. Imagine stress like a storm—without proper preparation, it can wreak havoc on your health. However, if you develop the right coping strategies, you can weather the storm with minimal disruption.

Incorporate stress-relieving activities into your daily routine, such as deep breathing exercises, meditation, or yoga. These practices calm your nervous system and reduce cortisol levels, helping to keep blood sugar in check. Even a few minutes of deep breathing or a short meditation session can make a big difference in how your body responds to stress.

Prioritize Sleep for Blood Sugar Balance
Sleep is one of the most underrated factors in blood sugar control, yet it's crucial for long-term balance. Poor sleep disrupts insulin sensitivity and increases hunger hormones, leading to higher blood sugar levels and cravings for sugary foods. Think of sleep as the body's natural reset button—when you don't get enough, your system doesn't function properly, and blood sugar regulation suffers.

Establish a consistent sleep routine to support glucose balance. Aim for 7-9 hours of sleep per night and create a relaxing bedtime routine that helps signal your body it's time to wind down. This could include dimming the lights, reading a book, or practicing gentle stretches. Avoid caffeine and screen time in the evening, as these can interfere with your ability to fall asleep and stay asleep. Prioritizing rest ensures your body is equipped to handle blood sugar regulation the next day.

Tracking Your Progress: Staying Accountable

Lastly, tracking your progress is key to sustaining lifelong habits. Monitoring your blood sugar levels regularly, either through finger-prick testing or using a continuous glucose monitor (CGM), allows you to see how your habits are affecting your glucose levels. Think of this as checking the dashboard of your car—without monitoring, you don't know if you're running low on fuel or need to make adjustments.

Keep a journal of your blood sugar readings, along with notes on your diet, physical activity, stress levels, and sleep. Over time, this information provides valuable insights into what works best for your body, allowing you to fine-tune your habits for optimal glucose balance. Tracking also keeps you accountable and motivated to stick with the behaviors that lead to success.

Conclusion: Building Habits for Lifelong Health

Creating sustainable habits for blood sugar balance is a long-term commitment, but the rewards are worth it. By starting small, personalizing your approach, and designing an environment that supports success, you can create lasting change. Incorporating mindful eating, regular movement, stress management, and prioritizing sleep all contribute to lifelong blood sugar balance. Stay consistent, track your progress, and celebrate the small victories along the way. These habits will not only help you manage your blood sugar but also enhance your overall well-being for years to come.

www.ingramcontent.com/pod-product-compliance
Lightning Source LLC
Chambersburg PA
CBHW061350250726
48657CB00004B/1415